Executive Functioning Workbook For Kids

Kid's Social, and Moral Development to Boost Positivity and Reduce Negativity Through Polishing Executive Skills.

By

Mary C. Norris

Kangaroo Publications

© **Copyright 2022 by Kangaroo Publications - All rights reserved.**

Without the prior written permission of the Publisher, no part of this publication may be stored in a retrieval system, replicated, or transferred in any form or medium, digital, scanning, recording, printing, mechanical, or otherwise, except as permitted under 1976 United States Copyright Act, section 107 or 108. Permission concerns should be directed to the publisher's permission department.

Legal Notice

This book is copyright protected. It is only to be used for personal purposes. Without the author's or publisher's permission, you cannot paraphrase, quote, copy, distribute, sell, or change any part of the information in this book.

Disclaimer Notice

This book is written and published independently. Please keep in mind that the material in this publication is solely for educational and entertaining purposes. All efforts have provided authentic, up-to-date, trustworthy, and comprehensive information. There are no express or implied assurances. The purpose of this book's material is to assist readers in having a better understanding of the subject matter. The activities, information, and exercises are provided solely for self-help information. This book is not intended to replace expert psychologists, legal, financial, or other guidance. If you require counseling, please get in touch with a qualified professional.

By reading this text, the reader accepts that the author will not be held liable for any damages, indirectly or directly, experienced due to the use of the information included herein, particularly, but not limited to, omissions, errors, or inaccuracies. As a reader, you are accountable for your decisions, actions, and consequences.

TABLE OF CONTENTS

A NOTE TO THE GROWN-UPS 5
HELLO, LITTLE THINKERS! 8
QUICK ROUND OF EXECUTIVE FUNCTIONING 10

CHAPTER 1 EXECUTIVE FUNCTION ZONES....................16
1.1 Active Memory..19
1.2 Adaptive Thinking..23
1.3 What Causes Slow Processing Speed? 24
1.4 Potential Root Causes of Executive Function Disorders 33

CHAPTER 2: SMART GOALS AND EXECUTIVE FUNCTIONING SKILLS 37
2.1 Goal Setting: A Fun Way to Develop Executive Function Skills 38
2.2 Planning...40
2.3 Organization 40
2.4 Time Management 40
2.5 Task Initiation 41
2.6 Working Memory..41
2.7 Metacognition 41
2.8 Self-Control 42

CHAPTER 3: APPROACHES TO LEARNING AND EXECUTIVE FUNCTIONING..45
3.1 Six Different Learning Strategies 47

CHAPTER 4: ACHIEVING EXECUTIVE FUNCTION IN CHILDREN 53

4.1 Providing Educator Support 53
4.2 Providing Ecological Support 57
4.3 Self- Surveillance 62

CHAPTER 5: BREAK THE NEGATIVITY LOOP 67
5.1 Start with Validating Feelings...73
5.2 The Three Varieties of Self-Control 76
5.3 Be Positive: Try Being Optimistic! 80
5.4 Develop Thankfulness: *Practice Being Thankful*......................84
5.5 Practical Approach and Frequently Asked Questions 85

OUTCOMES 93

A Note to the Grown-ups

In my memory, one parent-teacher meeting overtakes the rest. My spouse and I were at our son's fourth-grade classroom at the start of the academic year. The instructor said that the students had just finished a writing evaluation at the outset.

She stated, "They had twenty minutes to respond to a prompt.

Oh, our son is very imaginative. How did he fare?

She handed us a blank sheet of paper bearing our son's name. We were perplexed.

Didn't he write anything? I exclaimed in shock.

This child had a strong vocabulary and a creative imagination. At home, he would tell lengthy tales. In his writings, he would doodle and write about animals with eccentric personalities and superpowers but when asked to write an open-ended essay at school, he found himself at a loss for words.

Did he have a block on writing? Maybe it was just a poor day for him.

The instructor disagreed. She inhaled deeply. I did too! I continued to listen genuinely after that: "It's probable that your son felt overwhelmed by the increased demands of this writing assignment. Does he have executive function issues?

I looked at my spouse, and we both said, "Struggle with what?" That's how we came to understand executive functioning in kids and the significance of writing about it.

The ability to organize our thoughts and plan, which enables us to accomplish our goals, is ultimately developed by some mix of genes and life experiences, similar to how the theory of mind works. Infancy is the time when executive functioning development starts. Watch a baby learn that the figures on her mobile will revolve by kicking her legs. She will enjoy making things happen once she understands leg-kicking and mobile motion. She knows how to retain an idea in mind while working on completing a task ("kick to move mobile").

What occurs when children lack enough executive function?

Executive function is usually hampered in conditions like autism and ADHD. The poor executive function may account for a large portion of what we currently refer to as ADHD. Behavioral disorders, particularly those characterized by poor self-control, addiction, a lack of adequate restraint, and an inability to anticipate the effects of actions, are also categorized as executive function impairment.

Many kids (and adults), including some who perform well on cognitive tests but struggle for no apparent reason, might also lack executive function. In other words, sound future planning is impossible without vital executive function. Furthermore, without a solid executive function, there is little motivation to complete tedious tasks, like memorization and study, for possible future benefits.

So, how can I support my kid in developing his abilities?

There are strategies to assist kids in "getting their acts together," depending on the prime reasons for distractibility and other potential executive function deficits. Experts start by addressing attention concerns if, as is frequently the case, attention deficits cause and trigger the issue. Teachers and tutors frequently provide step-by-step assistance with time management, by utilizing checklists, due dates, planners, and to-do lists. It is helpful to enforce regularly planned cleanup times to keep the workspace orderly. Some children require careful, supportive guidance in the "clearing the decks" procedure to complete a project from start to finish. If your child consistently has problems with planning and organization, communicate with his teacher or the school psychologist about the best ways to support him.

The physical maturation of the brain occurs at varying speeds, even in children of the same age or grade. The ideal strategy, however long it takes, is to meet each child where he/she is and let steady progress and mastery win the day. Follow the example set by the kind professionals caring for your youngster. Discover the world and its difficulties through his/her eyes. Many kids have surmounted the challenge of poor executive function and succeeded in school, even if it took time and endless patience.

Hello, Little Thinkers!

Executive Functioning Skills: What are They?

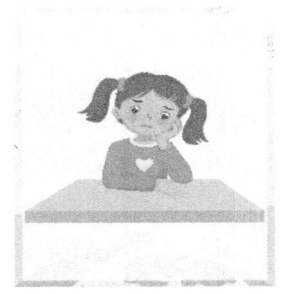

Young minds frequently ask themselves these issues, and with good cause. Our brains' executive functioning mechanisms enable us to carry out our daily duties. These include our capacity for task prioritization, material organization, activity focus, and grit under pressure. These abilities are crucial, which should go without saying. We put these abilities to practice frequently each day without even realizing it. Even while reading this book, you are engaging your attention, metacognition, and working memory.

We frequently don't even consider using these skills when they come naturally to us. You've trained your brain to use your talents when needed, which is lovely. Let's look at an illustration.

When you have a task to complete, you probably talk to yourself about starting it (task initiation), paying attention to it while ignoring distractions, and completing it (perseverance).

Every person has a different set of executive functioning strengths and challenges. Executive functioning issues might therefore affect different people in different ways. While specific actions may be overt, others may be subtler. It is helpful to look for patterns of behavior over time when identifying Executive Functioning (EF) challenges.

Children and teenagers with executive functioning issues may:

- *Have trouble starting or completing things.*

- *Regularly misplace or lose stuff.*
- *Face difficulty in organizing oneself or maintaining it.*
- *Forget the steps in a task's instructions.*
- *Have trouble concentrating on a job or switching between tasks.*
- *Take impulsive action (acting without thinking through a situation).*
- *Hastily complete the work before the deadline.*
- *Have trouble keeping track of time.*
- *Become irritated by scheduling modifications.*

Additionally, there is a wide range in the difficulty of the challenge. While some children can adjust to the schedule changes without getting upset, others find it impossible to carry on with their daily routines. Understanding each of your kids individually and their requirements become crucial in this situation because some children may only require simple accommodations while others require urgent interventions.

Quick Round of Executive Functioning

Almost everyone can gain executive function skills, although no one is born with them.

The higher-order cognitive abilities known as executive functions help kids control their behavior and engage in goal-oriented activities. Executive functions include being self-directed, avoiding distractions, being flexible, and connecting various concepts and ideas.

"High-level non-cognitive skills like resilience, curiosity, and academic tenacity are challenging for a child to acquire without first building a foundation of executive functions, a capacity for self-awareness, and relationship skills, according to Brooke Stafford-Brizard, and those abilities, in turn, are built upon a foundation of attributes cultivated during the formative years of life, such as a strong sense of attachment, the capacity for stress management, and self-control".

"There will be obstacles in the way of your goals. Every one of us has experienced them. But you don't have to let challenges stop you. Do not turn around and give up if you hit a wall. Find a way to scale, pass through, or maneuver around it."
Jordan, Michael

A typical day for a kid named Alex struggling with executive functioning...

Meet Alex, a sixth-grader with difficulties in executive functioning. He is nonetheless intelligent, even despite this. It indicates that his brain's self-management mechanism struggles to arrange and complete tasks. A crucial collection of mental abilities is the executive functions. Now, examine his day to understand how Alex's struggles with these abilities impact him at school and in his personal life.

Alex is aware of his forgetfulness. He has his cleats for the game today, I see. Running back inside to retrieve them, ultimately forgets his backpack there in haste to make the bus. He rushes through the school supply list that his mother had created for him. It's too late, though, as the bus is about to leave. He'll once again miss it.

Who has a solid response to the first question I gave you yesterday on the reading assignment from last night, asks Alex's teacher? Alex trembles in the hopes that he won't be pointed. The questions aren't in his planner, and he has no idea how to respond.

The lunch hour is the highlight of the school day. Alex, however, dominates the conversation by talking very loudly about his video games. He is unaware of his pals' increasing irritability.

In soccer, Alex is so intent on obtaining the ball that he neglects to remember which way he should be running once he has it. He rapidly runs to the nearest goal and promptly kicks the ball into his team's goal.

When Alex's mother orders him to turn off the television and set the table for supper, he is not pleased. When he assumes he is finished, his younger sister informs him that he once again forgot to provide each person with a cup. He loses his calm and yells at his sister out of frustration over losing his TV show.

After much nagging from his mother, Alex finally sits down to finish his homework but he is unsure about where to begin. When he searches the internet for a subject for his scientific report, due the following week, rather than working on the book report or the math problems due tomorrow, he pauses to play a video game.

When Alex does begin the book report, his thoughts are constantly bouncing about in his head. He struggles to find something to write and only manages to get one phrase down before giving up for the evening. Even though he has never accomplished anything when riding the bus with his pals, he believes that he can accomplish more tomorrow on the way to school.

His bedtime has long since passed. Alex is worn out. He tries to fall asleep, but his brain won't turn off. He keeps fretting that his book report will disappoint the teacher and that his teammates will make fun of him for kicking the ball into the wrong goal.

How Do You Define Executive Functioning Skills?
The cognitive, verbal, sensory, and motor skills accumulated over life to become successful adults are combined in executive functioning skills. We employ these abilities to carry out daily activities, such as playing, socializing, and learning, beginning at a very young age. Almost every element of our everyday lives uses executive function skills, but as we reach school age, these abilities play a crucial role.

As children of school age become more independent, they must learn practical time management skills to complete tests, assignments, and other tasks on schedule. They must pay attention to learning new things and maintain sufficient organization to locate the required resources.

How do Executive Functioning Capabilities Change with Age?
Many psychologists and child development specialists believe that all people are born with some genetic propensity or innate capacity to acquire behaviors related to executive functioning.

Then, through environmental learning, we build executive functioning abilities, many of which occur in the first two years of life. Children develop their executive functioning abilities through social play activities. We start to shoulder more responsibility at home and school between the ages of 5 and 12. Parents, educators, and other caregivers offer the opportunity for children to practice executive functioning skills throughout these activities and encourage them when they succeed. To assist kids in learning critical executive functioning activities like organization, time management, emotional regulation, and others, adults create a "scaffolding" of support. By the time we reach adolescence and early adulthood, we have had various experiences that have molded our abilities in various fields.

At this point, the adults around us start to take down the scaffolding and anticipate that teenagers and young adults will keep using executive functioning skills independently. Even though kids may still make mistakes, they can have fulfilling lives in their homes, schools, and interpersonal interactions if they have a strong foundation in executive functioning skills.

The executive function of many children who learn and think differently is problematic.
Children are intelligent despite these challenges. Children with different brains have trouble focusing, setting objectives, getting started, and staying on track. It includes daily tasks and activities like doing homework.

These types of difficulties are frequently misunderstood. People may believe that children are merely being lazy or incapable of doing more but youngsters with executive function issues can thrive with the correct assistance. There are many methods to assist at home and in the classroom. Children who get support can keep up with their schoolwork and become more organized. Additionally, it may make individuals feel less anxious and more self-assured.

Before Reading Further, let's Jot Down Your Reflection

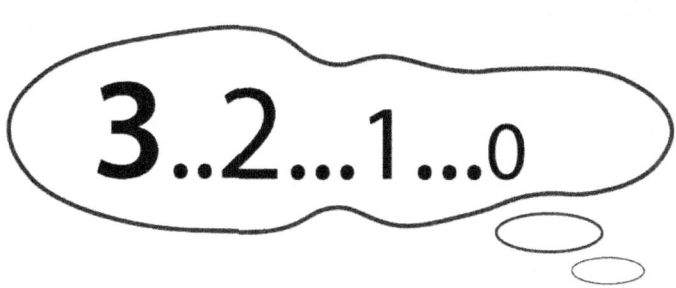

COUNTDOWN BY _____

3 things I know about...

2 questions I still have...

1 thing I will do...

Chapter 1 Executive Function Zones

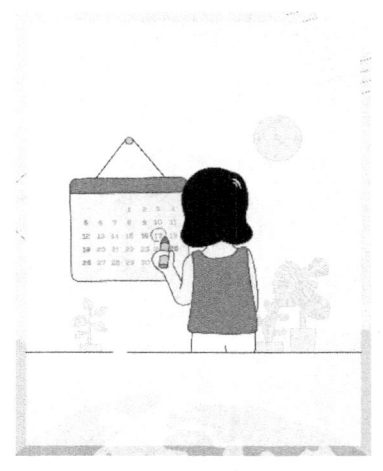

Children get a firmer understanding of their physical world as they progress from early infancy through primary school and acquire more organized and logical thinking skills. Executive function is one set of abilities that aids in this developmental process. Executive function abilities enable us to respond to inquiries like:

Why is it simpler for certain kids to get along with other kids?
Why are some situations more difficult for kids to control their emotions than others?
Why do some kids seem to have an easier time achieving their goals while others have trouble doing so?

How Does the Executive Functioning Occur?

Working memory, cognitive flexibility, and inhibitory control are the three cognitive processes that work together to form executive function. Children practice cognitive flexibility skills in primary school by working in teams or groups. For instance, to properly complete a task, a youngster may need to change from one thought to another and consider many options. A youngster can hold and retain many pieces of knowledge with working memory. Children in primary school, for instance, employ working memory when they have to recall numerous steps necessary to answer a challenging math problem. A youngster can stop an impulsive response and switch to one that is more appropriate for the situation, thanks to inhibitory control. When, for instance, they are eager and want to yell out a response to a question during a class discussion but choose to wait for their turn to speak instead, children employ inhibitory control skills. Children's behaviors show how these three cognitive processes interact and function in various ways. Executive function develops along with brain development and can be improved with time and effort. Children can plan and act in ways that help them become successful scholars, compassionate classroom citizens, and good friends as these skills develop.

- **Development of Executive Function**

Early in life, the executive function starts to develop. These abilities are influenced by maturity (including brain development) and interactions with adults in children's lives, such as parents, teachers, after-school caretakers, siblings, classmates, and extended family. In the setting of the early attachment relationship that infants have with their caregivers, the groundwork for executive function emerges. Babies are more likely to feel secure and safe when they engage with significant adults in their lives in a loving and supportive manner. Children gain confidence by experiencing security from dependable adults, enabling them to explore their surroundings easily, become independent, and practice problem-solving. Secure interactions also influence strong social and emotional development and executive function abilities in early childhood. Early executive function training increases a child's likelihood of exhibiting self-control in social and academic contexts, especially as they get older and move into more structured learning situations. Children's executive function abilities in elementary school can be shown in their ability to solve issues, staying on task, collaborating with others, and establishing friendships. Executive function abilities connect to academic success, social competence, and overall well-being, including physical and mental health.

- **Improving Executive Function Abilities**

For youngsters to develop their executive function, it's crucial to establish friendly and accommodating interactions with them. In particular, offering comfort to youngsters who are upset or in need of assistance aids in the scaffolding of executive function abilities. After stressful experiences, children should have a safe place to unwind. Numerous traits are shared by learning environments that promote the growth of strong executive function skills. These consist of the following:

- *Encouraging kids to keep an eye on their behavior*
- *The behavior of children should be expected.*
- *Arranged learning environments*

Consistent techniques of correction that emphasize teaching children about the consequences of their conduct include, setting limits without using punishment, and providing alternatives to incorrect behavior.

Executive function abilities can be improved, which is significant news. The best strategy to improve executive function skills is to incorporate them into regular activities, give kids chances to practice them in various situations, and provide encouraging feedback. To promote efficient executive function skills in primary school, the following are particularly crucial:

- *Creating an environment that is encouraging and helpful for all students*
- *Including opportunities for practicing executive function skills during academic study and social interactions*
- *Teaching educators how to demonstrate, emphasize and impart helpful executive function skills*
- *Encouraging teachers and after-school personnel to develop their effective executive function skills*
- *Assisting parents so that they can foster the development of their children's executive function at home*

The three main spheres of executive function are as follows:

1. Active memory
2. Adaptive thinking (also called flexible thinking)
3. Restraining power (which includes self-control)

1.1. Active Memory

One of the executive functions of the brain is working memory. It's a talent that enables us to work with knowledge without being sidetracked. Working memory can be compared to a temporary sticky note inside the brain. It secures new information so the brain can process it briefly and link it to existing knowledge.

Working memory, for instance, enables students to mentally "see" the numbers their teacher is stating in math class. They might not recall these numbers by the following class or even in ten minutes, but it's alright. Working memory has completed its short-term task by assisting individuals with the immediate task.

Working memory can be used over the long term as well. Additionally, it aids in the brain's organization of new data for long-term preservation. Working memory issues can cause the brain to store information in a disorganized way. Or it might not even store for a long time. Sometimes what appears to be a working memory problem is a problem with attention; the data was never entered into the brain's memory system in the first place.

Working memory and attention are essential for learning and daily activities. Both of these executive functioning components assist us in assimilating and comprehending new knowledge. However, despite their close connections, these functions are not the same. Here is a brief description of each one.

- **What is Attention?**

Our ability to absorb information is a function of attention. It also aids in the selection of pertinent data. Consider it like a funnel. It compiles the information that we require and transfers it to our brains. The art of paying attention well consists of four key components. Children may struggle with one or more of these elements.

Alertness: Children must be prepared to focus.

Selection: Children must be able to recognize what demands their attention. For instance, they must be able to concentrate on the teacher rather than the voices outside in the hallway.

Sustaining: Children must be able to sustain a modicum of attention throughout time. It might be for a 40-minute lecture or a three-minute presentation.

Shifting: Kids should be able to briefly shift their focus when significant new information is presented. They must be able to concentrate, for instance, on a quick announcement spoken over the intercom. They should then be able to focus their attention once more on the instructor.

> *Children who have attention problems might not remember what they have learned. It is because it never "went into their heads" initially.*

- **Working Memory Definition**

The attention funnel gathers information, which is then fed into the brain's short-term memory bank. It is an initial repository for new information. Experts refer to this procedure as "encoding." Additionally, this is where the brain shapes new knowledge to make it worthwhile. We refer to this process as "working memory."

Working memory is a dynamic and quick process. It enables us to apply newly acquired knowledge while engaged in an activity. Think about a social studies lecture. The teacher is discussing great explorers. As they listen, pupils' working memories process the information to give it context and meaning.

It frequently entails organizing bits of information in some way. That might be the chronological arrangement. Children may visualize Columbus on a timeline before Pizarro, for instance. They might even place Lewis and Clark's knowledge after Columbus. Children may classify what they are hearing or seeing. For instance, they might group explorers according to the nation they are from or the area they have explored.

Once this new knowledge has been processed, it is no longer stored in the brain's short-term memory. It then enters a more significant long-term "tank." At the end of the lecture, if the teacher gives the class a quiz, the material is taken from the long-term memory tank.
Children who struggle with working memory may have trouble organizing the knowledge they store in long-term memory. Due to improper packaging, it may not have much meaning. It might not be constructive as a result.

Information loss and failure to enter the long-term tank can be attributed to working memory problems.

Examples of Working Memory Issues

Here are some illustrations of how people with the troubling working memory appear.
- *Mental Arithmetic:* The teacher instructs the students to mentally add 21 and 13 before taking 6 out of the total. Children may recall the numbers that teacher instructed them to add: 21 and 13, but they won't remember what to do with them. Or, they might not keep track of the total (34), making it impossible to deduct six from it.

- *Observing Practical Guidelines:* People cannot remember every step when given a series of instructions, such as driving instructions. They might also forget the proper sequence.

- *Using Knowledge Afterward:* Some individuals could discover that the facts they have retained don't make sense. Problems with working memory prevent the brain from appropriately packaging the information in the first place.

Those who learn and think in unconventional ways struggle with working memory. In particular, this applies to children and people with ADHD. That's because executive function issues, such as poor working memory, are associated with ADHD.

1.2. Adaptive Thinking

Changing gears might be challenging for some children. They become agitated or irritated when their timetable is altered. They have trouble adjusting to change because there is only one conceivable schedule or solution that they can envision.

These young people have trouble with flexible thinking. Their struggles with coming up with new solutions to issues can have a significant influence on both learning and daily life. Children with troubled flexible thinking may become immobile in the face of a challenge. Alternatively, even if a strategy fails, they might keep trying it.

Conversations may contain instances of this restrictive way of thinking. Children might not comprehend, for instance, that certain words have several meanings. It can also manifest itself in academic work, such as when students utilize a math technique that only functions with a particular kind of word problem.

1.3. What Causes Slow Processing Speed?

When people have a slow processing speed, it takes them a long time to receive information, understand it, and react to it. The data may be represented visually, for as by letters or numbers. In addition, like spoken language, may be auditory. A sluggish cognitive speed can frequently provide difficulties at work, school, and social settings.

For instance, young children could find it challenging to acquire reading, writing, and counting fundamentals. People of all ages may struggle to complete activities precisely and promptly. They frequently struggle to retain new information.

It can be challenging to interact with other people. People with sluggish cognitive speeds could remain still for a short while before speaking. They could also take a while to explain anything. People's processing speeds—how rapidly they take in and utilize information—have nothing to do with their intelligence. Nevertheless, facing this obstacle can be very stressful and damage one's self-esteem.

- **Indications of Sluggish Processing**

Every aspect of life can be impacted by slow processing speed. It's a constant struggle, and the symptoms might change with age. You might still notice a few everyday things. People who digest information slowly might:

- *Become disoriented by a flood of information*
- *Need more time to decide or respond*
- *Miss social cues frequently*
- *Want the information to be read more than once to be understood*
- *Miss subtleties in discussion and find it difficult to follow*
- *Face difficulty adhering to rules and routines*
- *Feel it challenging to complete chores on schedule or within a fair time*

People can have trouble processing both visual and auditory information. However, they don't necessarily have problems with both. Others have trouble with motor speed. As a result, individuals find it difficult to respond rapidly to physical duties like filling out a form.

Executive Function Difficulties' Telltale Signs

Executive function issues can have a variety of effects on individuals. The issues frequently resemble ADHD symptoms. It is so because executive function is an issue with ADHD. Kids with organizational skill problems may find:

- *Difficulty starting and/or finishing tasks*
- *Trouble setting priorities*

- *Themselves forgetting what they just read or heard or have problems following a series of instructions.*
- *Problems in transferring their attention from one task to another and becoming highly emotional.*
- *Trouble organizing their thoughts and keeping track of their stuff.*
- *Difficulty in organizing their time*

Executive function issues are not diagnostic or a form of learning disability. However, those who learn and think in diverse ways are typical. Everybody who has ADHD struggles with it. Additionally, many individuals with learning difficulties also struggle with executive function.

- **Why do Some Kids Perform Actions Out of Sequence? Problems with Sequencing**

It is not logical. You've often explained to your youngster how to set the table: placemats first, then napkins, and forks on top of the napkins, but, your kid continues to query about the correct sequence. This may also be experienced with other tasks. It appears relatively simple to follow straightforward procedures in the proper order. Why is your youngster unable to understand what comes first, second, and third in a process? Learn more about sequencing issues and how you may assist your child in developing this ability.

- **How do Sequencing Issues Look Like?**

Sometimes we all forget to complete the processes in the proper order. We become preoccupied and make mistakes like adding the eggs to the pan before the butter. However, we do know the proper sequence and can explain how to make eggs to others.

Not all children are aware of sequencing and that can affect children in all facets of life, including school, athletics, interpersonal interactions, and careers after finishing school.

Not following directions is different from not following the stages in the right order. The task is incomplete or wrongly done. This implies that following the proper order of events is problematic. The difficulties manifest in various ways. Children may not follow the proper steps to solve an arithmetic issue in class. In social settings, they could tell convoluted or challenging-to-understand stories. When fixing anything at work, they may provide the tools to their boss in the wrong sequence.

Language is the first thing that children learn to order. Thus, early warning indications of problems frequently emerge as children learn to talk. For instance, a young child may say "milk I want" rather than "I want milk." Using the incorrect terse of a term after kindergarten, such as "I went to the store," could be a warning. Or, if children mix up the words in a phrase, they can say, "Mommy went to the store yesterday, and afterward, I got a ball". As kids age, that challenge manifests itself in ways other than language. Children also struggle with organizing their ideas and activities.

- **What Causes Sequencing Issues?**

Children have difficulty performing tasks in the proper order for a variety of reasons. They might not have first paid heed to the instructions. Or they could struggle to recall them. Another factor to consider is general organizational complexity. Children that struggle with these abilities, also referred to as executive functions, frequently struggle with sequencing. Kids with ADHD are included in this.

It's a processing issue for some kids. They might require extra time to process and comprehend the instructions. Other children might struggle to follow directions because of linguistic barriers.

- **How to Assist Your Youngster with Sequencing?**

Your child can benefit from your assistance in practicing step-by-step execution. Participate in joint activities that require sequencing. These include preparing food, doing laundry, and gardening. As you complete the task, explain it to your child and have them explain the sequential steps you took.

Talk about the movies or TV series you've seen. Ask your youngster to recount the story or a specific scene. It is also possible with books. Help your child organize things if they cannot identify a distinct beginning, middle, and end. Give a visual representation of the steps. Consider utilizing a graphic chart or a checklist that details each step needed to complete a task without asking what to do or when your youngster can check it before or during an activity.

For writing, use graphic organizers. Older children can practice writing and speaking stories with all the elements in the right order through these easy tools. Learning challenges may result from these issues. However, they don't imply that individuals are stupid or lazy. People with executive function issues are just as intelligent and diligent in their work as everyone else.

- **Differences in Learning and Thinking that Interfere with Time Management**

Not every child learns how to manage their time in the same way. Some children need more time to acquire abilities like anticipating needs and keeping track of details. Some young people might catch up with their peers on their own. Others require more assistance to succeed, such as children who learn and think in different than normal ways. Kids may improve their time management skills with the proper encouragement and lots of practice.

- **How Do Executive Function Issues Affect Time Management?**

How it works: A group of mental capacities is called executive functions. The brain uses these abilities to organize and process information. These abilities help children to plan, organize, get going, and stay on track. A key component of executive function is flexible thinking. Working memory is also a component of it. Our capacity for working memory allows us to retain new information so that we can use it later.

The link between time management: Kids who have trouble with these abilities frequently get distracted. For instance, poor working memory makes it challenging to retain knowledge long enough to plan and finish tasks.

How does ADHD Impact Time Management?

How it works: Focus and self-control are impacted by ADHD, a prevalent disorder. It is strongly related to executive functioning.

The relationship between ADHD and time management: Children with ADHD struggle with executive function and time management abilities. Time management issues might also arise from other ADHD symptoms. Things like difficulty focusing and sitting motionless are key exhibits.

The Impact of Dyscalculia on Time Management

How it works: A learning disability called dyscalculia makes it challenging to comprehend mathematical ideas and numbers.

The link to time management: Children with dyscalculia might struggle to read the time. They could also have trouble estimating how long the tasks will take. For instance, most children can "feel" how much time they have left when a teacher gives the class 20 minutes to do a quiz. It might be challenging for dyscalculic children to pace themselves since they may not know how much time they have left.

Time management issues might also result from other learning deficits. For instance, a youngster with dyslexia can take three times as long as other kids to read a novel. Children who struggle to write also struggle to take notes fast. Children with difficulty in school could also feel frustrated by things that are difficult for them. As a result, they may put off or procrastinate accomplishing things. It may also affect time management.

There are numerous techniques to assist your child in mastering time management, regardless of what is holding them back. Look for trends in the things that challenge your youngster. Inquire with the teacher to see if any related incidents occur at the school. Your youngster can improve time management skills with your aid if you search for the most satisfactory solutions together.

TIME MANAGEMENT
Urgent, Important...It can wait!

What are some things you need to get done? What's urgent, what's important, and what can wait? Use this worksheet to help you prioritize what you need to do!

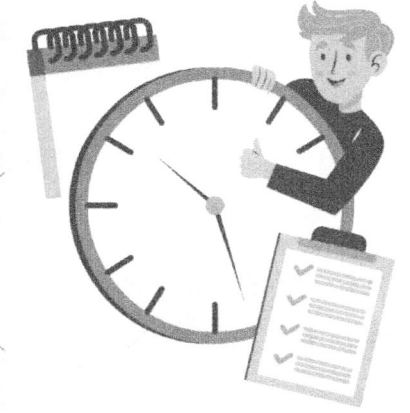

What are some things that need to get done as soon as possible?

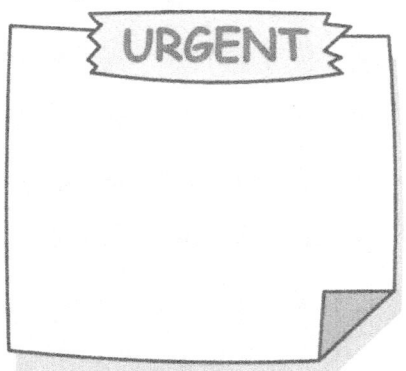

URGENT

What are some important things that need to get done, but not right way?

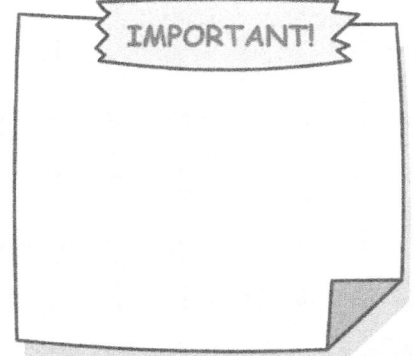

IMPORTANT!

What are some things on your list that that aren't urgent or important and can wait a few days?

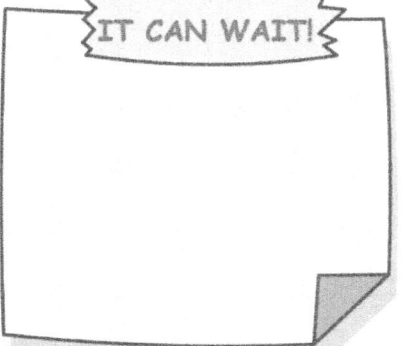

IT CAN WAIT!

Let Me Wish ……

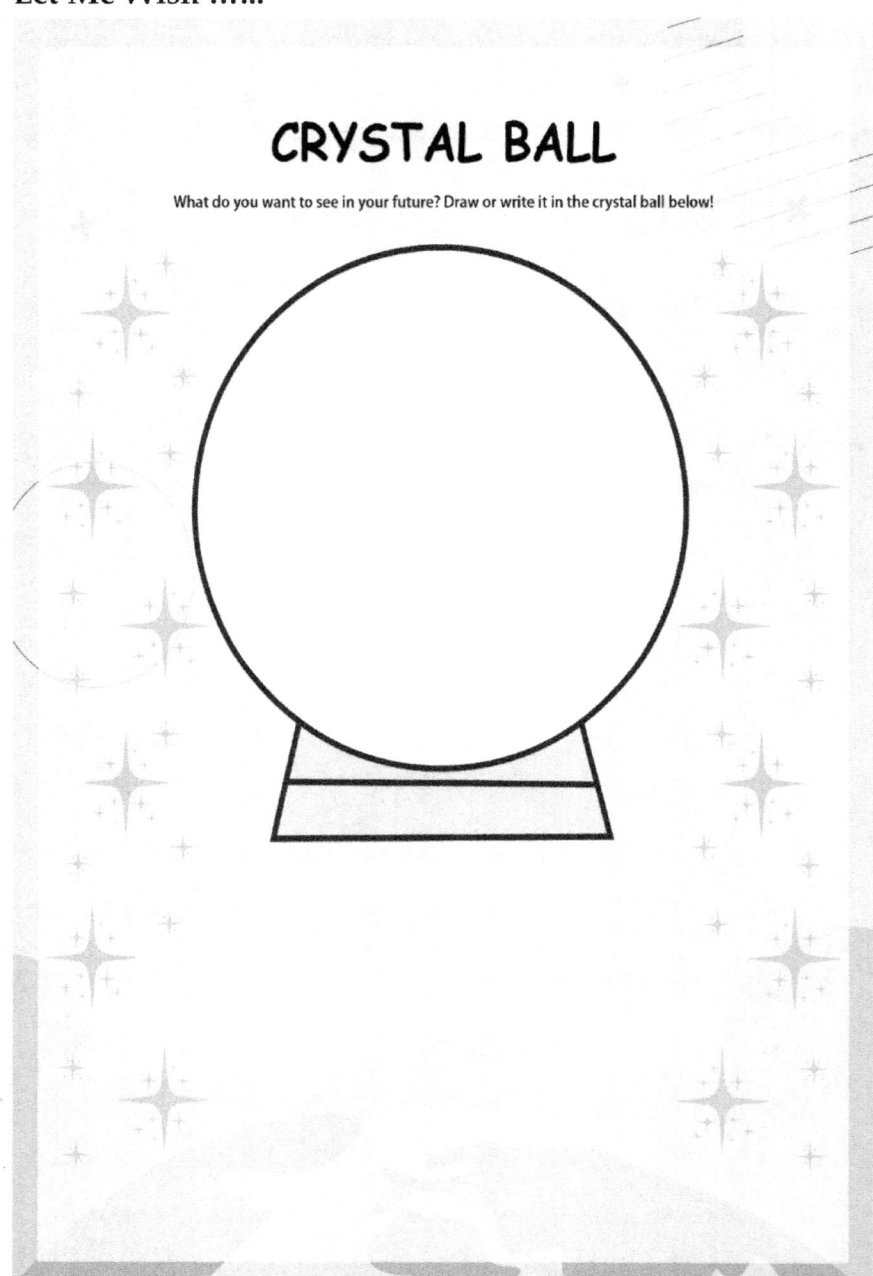

1.4. Potential Root Causes of Executive Function Disorders

"Attention deficit hyperactivity disorder (ADHD), a condition, affects how people act. People who have ADHD may seem antsy, have trouble focusing, and act impulsively.

Extensive research has been done on what impairs executive function and contributes to ADHD. Here are the two main elements:

1. **Variations in brain growth:** Researchers have studied the brain's executive function. They've discovered that those who struggle with executive function have a slower rate of development in specific brain regions. These regions are in charge of working memory and emotional regulation.
2. **Heredity and genes:** Family members of those who struggle with executive function are frequently also affected.

Additionally, difficulties in executive function frequently accompany learning difficulties. Executive function issues are not usually present in learning impairments. However, it's not unusual for kids with dyslexia or dyscalculia, to struggle with executive function. Executive function is not impaired by slow processing speed. However, it can lead to problems.

1.5. Executive Function Issues Diagnosis and Treatment

The term "executive function disorder" is a misnomer. However, there are specific exams that examine a variety of executive skills.

Among these abilities are:

- *Control of attentional inhibition*
- *Active memory*
- *Planning and organization*
- *Idea generation*
- *A set shift (the ability to shift from one task to another)*
- *Creation of ideas and words*

A thorough evaluation that considers many aspects of learning and thinking should include testing. Psychologists frequently provide these free examinations for schools. However, other categories of specialists also carry out this kind of testing. ***Some of the professionals provide the following therapies and methods:***

- **Cognitive Behavioral Treatment and Behavior Therapy (CBT)**
Positive behavior replacements are encouraged through behavior therapy. CBT aids in behavior management and thinking and emotion processing in children.
- **Medications**
There are drugs for ADHD, but none precisely for executive function.
- **Services for Schools**
School psychologists can collaborate with teachers to assist children in developing social skills and behavior management techniques. Special education teachers may help children to develop their organizational, social, and academic skills. They might also focus on behavior management techniques.
- **Coaching for Organizing**

You can hire these consultants. They are not academic skill-building tutors. They only focus on developing organization and time management abilities in kids, instead.

Doctor Here ………

Temper-ature

1. Using the thermometer. Color the thermometer in red to show how you feel when nobody wants to play with you.

2. List 3 feeling words to show how you feel.

_____

_____

_____

3. Identify 3 things you could do that would make you feel better.

_____

_____

_____

_____

_____

Chapter 2: Smart Goals and Executive Functioning Skills

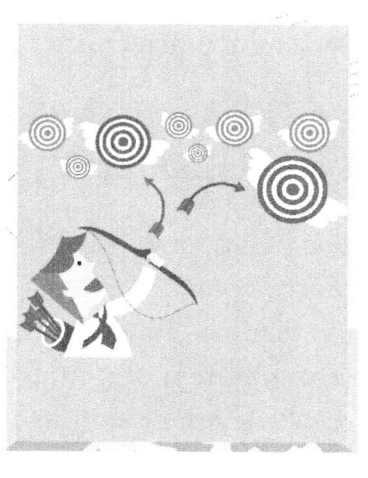

The activist, novelist, humorist, and physicist Benjamin Franklin once said, "For every minute spent organizing, an hour is earned.

Early in life, the evolution of executive function starts. These abilities are influenced by maturity (including brain development) and interactions with adults in children's lives, such as parents, teachers, after-school caretakers, siblings, classmates, and extended family. In the setting of the early attachment relationship that infants have with their caregivers, the groundwork for executive function emerges. Babies are more likely to feel secure and safe when they engage with significant adults in their lives in a loving and supportive manner. Children gain confidence by experiencing security from dependable adults, enabling them to explore their surroundings easily, become independent, and practice problem-solving. Social solid, secure interactions influence early childhood emotional development and executive function abilities. Early executive function training increases a child's likelihood of exhibiting self-control in social and academic contexts, especially as they get and move into more structured learning situations. Children's executive function abilities in elementary school can be shown in their ability to solve issues, stay on task, collaborate with others, and establish friends. Executive function abilities are essential to academic success, social competence, and overall well-being, including physical and mental health.

2.1. Goal Setting: A Fun Way to Develop Executive Function Skills

The behaviors necessary to plan and accomplish goals are made more accessible by having vital executive functioning. Expertise in flexible thinking, planning, self-monitoring, self-control, working memory, time management, and organizing are among the essential abilities associated with executive function. Although development starts in early childhood, these competencies are crucial for a child's growth and capacity for learning, and they continue to advance well into adulthood. Many executive function difficulties could indicate a learning difference, like ADHD or dyslexia.

Executive Functioning Skills

Executive Functioning encompasses a wide range of skills that help us organize our behavior, effectively complete tasks, and engage socially with others.

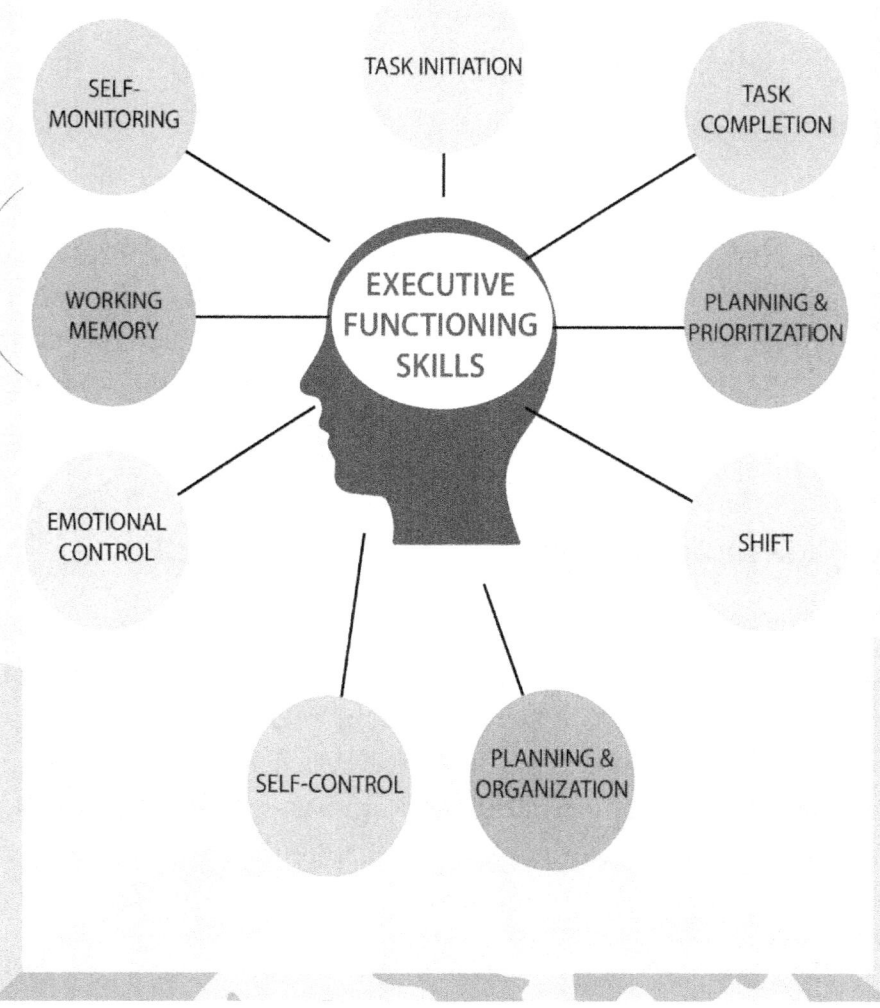

2.2 Planning

A child's capacity for planning, prioritizing various tasks, and thinking about the future are all excellent indicators of cognitive growth. A child with planning skills may develop a list of actions to complete a task and can accurately decide the most crucial components. Making a packing list, providing instructions, or composing a recipe are a few instances of planning.

2.3 Organization

An organization ability is a youngster's capacity to efficiently arrange objects or ideas in an ordered manner. Being organized helps children learn to tell stories clearly and keep track of their belongings, which is crucial for their growth and development. When a youngster chooses a separate folder or notepad for each academic subject or constantly follows any systematic procedure, it shows efficient organization.

2.4 Time Management

The ability of a youngster to create an effective schedule, complete tasks on time, and use patience while working on schoolwork is referred to as time management. Children need to understand how to manage time because it helps them switch between things more efficiently and increases their productivity, timeliness, and goal-setting skills. Effective time management is demonstrated when a multi-step task is completed before the deadline without rushing or sacrificing quality.

2.5 Task Initiation

When you look at their intended purpose, do you find most of your child's troublesome behaviors related to fleeing and avoiding tasks? Do you frequently need to nag your child to start tasks, even those that are simple to complete? Does your kid get sidetracked easily? Do you frequently require guidance from friends and family to find solutions on your own? If the answer is "positive," your child may require assistance with task starts. Task initiation refers to a child's capacity to develop ideas, solve issues, and respond to tasks independently. It's one of the fundamental executive functioning abilities, and many kids with attention- and ASD-related illnesses may struggle with it.

2.6 Working Memory

Working memory refers to a child's capacity to remember and store information to use later. Given that it is in charge of short-term memory and execution; this ability is essential for a youngster to succeed in the classroom. A child who successfully recalls and performs the directions for a step-by-step drill in gym class demonstrates a strong working memory.

2.7 Metacognition

A child with adaptable thinking skills can solve problems, adapt to circumstances, and get through immediate challenges. This ability also pertains to a child's capacity to consider other people's viewpoints. A child demonstrating this kind of cognitive thinking is not perplexed by common obstacles or disagreements. A young person who hits a roadblock while walking to school and comes up with a different route for the next time illustrates adaptive thinking.

2.8 Self-Control

The ability of a youngster to manage their physical or emotional outbursts is referred to as self-control. Impulse control prevents children from responding or acting without thinking. In contrast, emotional control enables them to maintain their composure and avoid the impulse to shut down or overreact in the face of setbacks or challenges. When a youngster obtains a poor grade on a test, but keeps their composure, and takes in constructive feedback, while remaining level-headed and learning from their mistakes, this also illustrates successful self-control in executive function.

Windowpane - Note-Taking

Name: _____ Date: _____

Important Words and Definitions	
Important Dates	Important Events
Summary of Learning	Rating of my learning: ◄─────────────► Unsure　　　　　　Got it Questions I Have

Tell Us What Makes You Smile

Name: _____ Date: _____

Simile Summary

A.. is like a ....
because...

Chapter 3: Approaches to Learning and Executive Functioning

> *How can we assist kids in making sense of the world they are about to enter?*

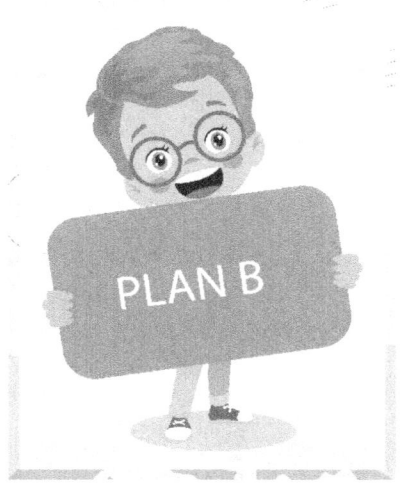

Every generation has asked about this issue as they have watched their children go from school to the workplace. It has lasted from our rural beginnings, the Industrial Revolution, international conflicts, and till today, the age of technological innovation.

Every generation has increased the complexity and integration of the skills that our children are required to possess, putting an increasing amount of strain on schools, particularly in light of the internet's role in the explosion of knowledge. Information is now more easily accessible on a global scale than it has ever been. A platform for understanding the world around us, developing original thoughts, ideas, and opinions, questioning the status quo, or extending the thinking of others, approaches to learning are some of the chances for lifelong learning. They consist of five crucial trans-disciplinary abilities:

1. Thinking

Critical Thinking: How do you analyze and assess problems and concepts? How can you come up with original ideas and consider new viewpoints?

Transfer Skills: In what situations can you apply your knowledge and skills?

2. Communication

How can you learn to read, write, and utilize language? How can you appropriately interact to communicate ideas, messages, and information?

3. Research

Information Literacy Skills: How can you discover, interpret, and produce information? How can you use and create ideas and information through media interaction? What level of media literacy do you possess?

4. Social

Collaboration Techniques: What are some effective teamwork techniques?

5. Self-management

Organizational Skills: What time and task management techniques do you use?

Affective Skills: How can you control your emotions?

Reflection Techniques: How can you (re)evaluate the learning process?

The word "*learning strategy*" is very self-explanatory. A learning approach is any strategy that you employ to acquire knowledge. These skills are timeless and help us handle the information and obstacles presented to us every day, regardless of age or experience in school or the workplace. Here, a learning technique is classified according to the objectives it aids in achieving. Therefore, if a learning strategy has been shown to aid in fact memorization, it will be characterized entirely in light of this attribute rather than how the brain functions, how knowledge is kept, or any other scientific explanation.

The child is asked to choose a teaching strategy that complements the executive learning objectives. Makes sure that the process works as intended. Regardless of the child's preferred learning style, each method of instruction is most effective for the particular purpose and fits them perfectly.

3.1. Six Different Learning Strategies

Since there are no set boundaries for learning, it is only proper that different learning methodologies exist to correspond with different executive learning objectives. It is vital to be informed of all your possibilities to pick the one that best suits your goals.

1. Behavioristic Approach

This method will be pretty simple for you to comprehend if you are familiar with the behaviorism theory of learning. As the name implies, this strategy focuses primarily on behavior. This method works best for learning anything that is intended to alter behavior.

Several talents necessitate a shift in behavior as opposed to information retention. It is mainly employed in practical education.

- **Repetition** and **reinforcement:** *are critical components of the behavioristic learning strategy.*
- **Recognition:** *When learners recognize something, they receive a signal of new information or an occurrence.*
- **Stimulus:** *The child responds to the knowledge they have been given.*
- **Multiple discrimination:** *In this type of learning, the child responds, but the replies are carefully selected to be the most pertinent to the information received.*
- **Concept learning:** *The child understands the meaning rather than the information based on the stimulus that the information activates.*

- ***Linguistic chain learning:*** *The learner connects new information with a specific verbal pattern based on the information they have received.*
- ***Motor chain learning:*** *In this kind of learning, the learner performs a series of steps they believe to be necessary.*
- ***Developing rules:*** *is a progression from conceptual learning when the child acts by what they have understood by forming mental rules.*
- ***Problem-solving:*** *The child formulates guidelines after grasping the idea, then uses all the knowledge at hand to produce something original.*

Technically, these categories characterize the behaviors that any new information may inspire.

2. Social Learning

Social learning and the behavioristic approach are closely related. In actuality, it is a development of the same idea. Instead of concentrating on the child's behavior, the social learning strategy entails observing the behaviors of others. Children, for instance, often imitate what they observe their parents doing. This method also highlights the idea that kids learn best by doing, regardless of their age or surroundings.

3. A Constructive Strategy

The constructivist learning approach is focused on building foundational knowledge. This method should practice skills that demand the child to be creative. Reflection and reevaluation are given a lot of attention in this technique. Forging associations and connections between new information and ancient knowledge in their minds enable the learner to brainstorm. It also gives the learner control over the direction that their education will go in.

4. Cognitive Strategy

Memorization and retention are the main goals of the cognitive learning approach. Do not interpret this as a method of information cramming. Instead, it uses a deep approach that enables the brain to comprehend and retain the data over time.

It is an excellent learning method for anything that requires memorizing larger chunks of material. However, you should also ensure that you fully comprehend all the information ingrained in your mind.

5. Experience-Based Method

The experiential learning method is used when you learn something by really doing it. Different types of encounters can teach children different things. It could involve observing an event, taking part in it, deliberately trying out a new technique, or thinking back on any of these experiences. In any case, the child must play a significant role in the experience. This results in first-hand education.

6. Humanist Perspective

The idea of kindness for all is the cornerstone of humanistic theory. It aspires to a peaceful, united world in which knowledge is evenly distributed and children acquire abilities and knowledge that have good impacts.

You may have figured by now that this strategy performs best when applied to collaborative projects. With this method of instruction, learning that has spiritual underpinnings or is community-focused will be done correctly. This method begins by urging the child to concentrate on what is correct instead of wrong.

Also, there are two variations of the humanistic approach:

The simplest form of learning is the transmission of knowledge or pedagogy but andragogy adds appeal by giving children complete control over their education.

Therefore, this approach works well for highly motivated learners who dislike being in charge.

How does a child use various learning strategies?

How can a child employ these learning strategies, then?

Well, child, hold the wheel now. Any of the methods can be applied wherever children feel they fit best but, to help kids understand what works best in which situation, here are a few examples:

- *Behavioristic Strategy*

Anything involving behavior can be taught using this method. Enhance children's emotional stability, work on controlling anger, or learn other self-help techniques.

- *Social Development*

There are many situations in this life where interacting with others is necessary. Any ability falling within this category is best learned through social learning.

- *Constructivist Methodology*

The constructivist learning approach is helpful for creative abilities.

- *Cognitive Method*

This method is excellent for research because it focuses on memory-intensive activities.

- *Experience-Based Method*

This learning strategy should be used to tackle anything that calls for a practical perspective.

- *Humanistic Method*

Any ability can be taught using the humanistic approach; the only distinction is that the children are mainly in charge. Therefore, the best abilities to learn with this method are those through which the person is highly motivated to learn. For community-based or spiritual learning, it works even better.

With this method, children can learn anything — from cooking to computing to calligraphy — as long as kids are willing to take action and be accountable!

Let's Observe Your Behavior

Behavior Change Plan
What behavior do I want to change?

☆ _____ ☆

What will happen if I no longer do this behavior? _____

_____

What can I do to start preparing to change?

1. _____
2. _____
3. _____

What steps do I need to take to make these changes happen?

1. _____
2. _____
3. _____

What can other people do to help me change my behavior?

1. _____
2. _____
3. _____

How will I know that I'm making progress? _____

_____

What should I do if I start to go backwards? _____

_____

What is something I can do today to start changing my behavior? _____

_____

Chapter 4: Achieving Executive Function in Children

Not all children develop their executive functions to the same degree. These underachievers may benefit from additional support in the classroom and at home as they work to improve their executive function.

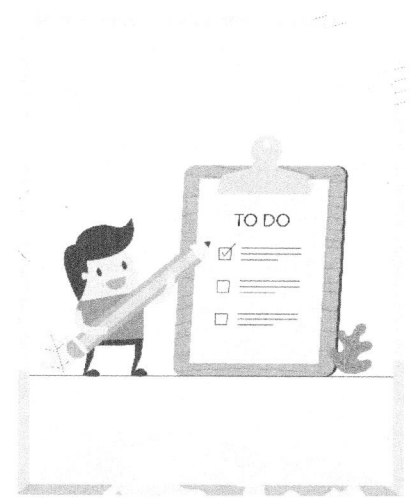

4.1. Providing Educator Support

One must first determine the kind of deficit; the learner is experiencing to address a certain deficit. Lack of knowledge prevents a child from knowing what to do or how to complete a task. For instance, active listening should be taught by citing examples to children who struggle to control their desires to speak while others are speaking. Teachers might also draw a diagram showing pupils' active listening looks and sounds.

While children may understand how to execute a task, they could struggle to determine when and how to use the necessary abilities. The teacher may verify that a child with this deficit has all the necessary supplies to do a task. The instructor could supply a list of the required supplies. For more advanced kids, the teacher might request that they make a list first before collecting the necessary supplies.

Metacognition: Using metacognitive language is another method for resolving executive function deficiencies. For instance, explaining the challenge to a child might be helpful. *You're lacking a pencil, I notice. To finish the project, you will need a pencil. Where might one be located in the classroom?*

It can be beneficial to demonstrate the procedures or inquiries children could make for themselves in the classroom to encourage independence with a skill. Kids can repeat instructions to a companion before asking a volunteer to repeat them to the class as a whole. Although it doesn't take much time, this procedure gives children who might require more time for auditory processing and repetition.

Posting schedules can be a helpful tool in learning time management techniques. A daily classroom plan helps children prepare for the following activities. A time block is divided into smaller segments by an activity schedule, specifying how each period will be used and the sequence in which activities will be offered. These timetables are frequently posted so all children can access them during the school day.

Long-term projects might be particularly difficult for kids who have executive function issues. Teaching kids directly how to organize more significant projects and divide them into smaller, more manageable chunks, is one way to solve this problem. Place the smaller benchmark targets on the calendar along with the dates by which each micro assignment will be completed.

Before beginning new learning: Give children the chance to review prior knowledge. The review may take the form of a brief oral presentation, or teachers may have children share their memories of the previous day in pairs.

Another format for a review may be a mind map or concept map developed in small groups. Concept maps are effective visual note-taking, contrasting/comparison, and writing tools. Since, organizing thoughts can be just as challenging as managing time and materials, graphic organizers might be especially beneficial for kids with executive function deficiencies.

Interaction with teachers: Teachers' actions significantly impact helping children who might struggle with executive function. Kids with deficiencies should receive frequent teacher check-ins, offering individualized guidance when necessary. Additionally, exhibiting compassion and employing constructive criticism with deficit-ridden children might enhance their academic experience.

4.2. Providing Ecological Support

Supporting the environment entails establishing an environment where kids can flourish. Some quick techniques for assisting pupils in enhancing executive function include:

Publish your Daily Schedule: Child-centered routines and processes provide structure. Offer visual aids, such as timetables and folders with color-coded schedules and posters with routines or methods for fixing problems. Consider underlining essential phrases and concepts in texts. Reduce clutter and provide distinct locations for each child in the classroom.

Possibility for Growth

It takes time for the executive function to develop fully, and every child develops it at a different rate. The human brain's prefrontal cortex is constantly developing and changing in young children and adolescents. Through classroom tactics and support, children with deficiencies in executive functions can develop; thanks to the human brain's incredible ability to learn.

- *What Would Occur if a Youngster Had Impaired Executive Function?*

Children with low executive function often develop into adults with poor executive function if they do not acquire specific executive functioning skills as they grow older. An adult who didn't submit a work project on time because they failed to jot down the deadline any of the four times their supervisor reminded them is likely to be a youngster who forgot where they placed their homework, let alone what the actual assignment was. Given this relationship, it is easy to comprehend why early development of adequate executive function skills is essential for success in the future.

- *How to Improve the Executive Functions of Your Child?*

Executive function issues, such as difficulties automating or planning, are a defining feature of ADHD. And that can rapidly become quite annoying. Parents, use these suggestions to strengthen each of the seven executive functions and aid in your child's independence.

- *Executive Dysfunction: A Better Understanding*

Executive function issues, including trouble automating tasks or planning, are hallmarks of ADHD. And that can start to bother you pretty fast. Follow these parenting tips to help your child become more independent while strengthening the seven executive functions.

1. Make Accountability Mandatory

Many parents are confused about how much responsibility is appropriate. ADHD is a timing issue more than a lack of awareness of consequences. The following steps can help your child's executive functioning, but the first thing you shouldn't do is free her of responsibility. Make her more accountable instead; expecting her to finish the required chores may show your faith in her abilities.

2. Jot it down

To overcome the limitations of working memory, make information visible using note cards, signs, sticky notes, lists, journals, or anything else. When the content is right in front of your child, it will be easier to encourage his executive functions and help him improve his working memory.

3. Externalize time

Make time a concrete, quantifiable concept by using one of the various clocks, timers, counters, or programs that are accessible. Helping your child comprehend how much time has passed, how much time still has to pass, and how quickly it is passing is a great way to counteract the common ADHD issue of "time blindness."

4. Share Incentive

Use rewards to externalize incentives. Someone with executive function difficulties may struggle to find the motivation to complete tasks that don't have immediate rewards. Creating fake motivating mechanisms like token systems or daily report cards is desirable in these situations. A child's motivation increases when short-term rewards are utilized to reinforce long-term goals.

5. Encourage hands-on learning

Give them command of the circumstance! Kids can reconcile their verbal and non-verbal working memories and improve their executive functions by making math problems as tangible as feasible. Examples include teaching simple addition and subtraction with jelly beans or colored blocks or practicing sentence construction with word magnets.

6. Stop to recharge

Executive and self-regulation skills are limited in number. If your child works too hard for too short of a period, they could quickly become exhausted (like while taking a test). When your child is involved in activities that drain their organizational system, encourage regular breaks, so they have a chance to refuel. Breaks can provide your child the energy they need to finish a task without getting distracted or losing attention when they last between three and ten minutes.

7. Start practicing the motivational talk

Do you remember the pre-game pep talk in the locker room? Your child requires one every day and sometimes more frequently. You should have your child practice saying, "You can do this," to help her develop her self-confidence. Children who speak highly of themselves are inspired to work harder and get closer to their goals. Visualizing success and mentally doing the required steps is a fantastic method for recharging the system and enhancing planning abilities.

8. Physical Activities

Exercise has several well-known benefits, one of which is a rise in your child's executive functioning. Over the week, regular exercise can help him refuel (and possibly expand his tank!) and control his ADHD symptoms more effectively. To exercise, try joining a group activity, attending a regular park playdate, or going for an impromptu run in the backyard.

9. Show sympathy

It's a huge one, people. Most of the time, individuals with ADHD are just as intelligent as their peers, but they cannot display their knowledge due to difficulties with executive function. The key to treatment is altering their surroundings to support them. To help children learn, it is crucial that the people in their lives, especially their parents, exhibit empathy. If your child does something wrong, wait a moment before yelling at them. Think about what went wrong and how you can help him learn from his mistake.

10. Communication

Make it clear to the child that you believe in him or her and want them to succeed. Unfortunately, a child will frequently fail if we anticipate them to struggle. Conversely, a child will frequently succeed if we expect them to succeed. Children frequently internalize our expectations of them, so their expectations may be realized. What if, for example, we told children with ADHD that a particular test has been designed to be ADHD-friendly and that, on this particular test, individuals with ADHD score equally well as people without ADHD, if not higher? What if we assured children that they will succeed in adulthood and that having ADHD is a positive because x, y, and z?

- Giving them responsibilities will show them that you believe in them and make them feel significant.
- Reiterate the ideas that everyone makes errors and that growth requires learning from them.

Think about your advantages

Identify doable challenges: Gaining mastery of a difficult task inspires pride, assurance, and joy. Kids can overcome challenges regularly through sports and other activities by working hard and practicing. The difficulties must be surmountable, though.

Show tolerance: You might feel anxious if you're constantly rushing. Give people the time and space to find solutions on their own.

Promote your child's physical, emotional, social, and spiritual well-being: These elements influence one another and are inextricably linked

4.3. Self- Surveillance

Self-monitoring is a fancy technique you frequently employ to maintain tabs on your activities. You make several judgments as you go along: What's the status of the activity? What's effective and what isn't? Should I change anything? For instance, when preparing breakfast, you first ensure the butter in the pan has melted before adding the eggs. You could ask yourself, "What do I need to do differently this time?" if the eggs were runny the last time.

The same ability also applies to learning. Kids use these four techniques to monitor their learning.

- *Self-Monitoring and Fundamental Education*

Self-monitoring is a tool used by children to study subjects like math and reading. They also use it for more fundamental tasks like following instructions, remembering deadlines, and reviewing work.

Your youngster may not catch problems when editing a paper or checking for math errors if she has strong self-monitoring abilities. She might also find it difficult to judge whether she is correctly following instructions. Knowing when she needs to seek assistance can be challenging as a result.

- *Math and Self-Monitoring*

Kids utilize self-monitoring when it comes to math to decide how to approach a problem and assess whether their solution makes sense. Younger children use it to select the operation (or operations) to apply to a word problem. If your kid has trouble with this skill, you could notice that she has trouble interpreting hint terms (such as how much less than or in addition to) or deciding whether to use the + or - sign when she writes the problem.

Older children can use self-monitoring to check their solutions by applying the opposite action, such as multiplying, to check a division issue. Children utilize the skill of self-monitoring to check that they have completed all of the steps in a problem and that each component was completed appropriately. If your child has troubled self-monitoring, she can perform any or all steps incorrectly without being aware. She might not be aware that the answer is illogical.

- *Self-Awareness and Reading Instruction*

Decoding is a beginning reader's process to check whether the sounds she's using for the letters fit together to form a word she recognizes. Children who self-check are more likely to go back and reconsider a term when they feel it doesn't sound correct.

Your youngster might not recognize it doesn't make sense if she reads the word boat as bow-AT due to self-monitoring difficulties. As she advances and starts to read sentences, she might experience a similar difficulty discerning which word makes sense in that situation and determining which one doesn't.

- *Self-Monitoring and Comprehension of Text*

Self-monitoring helps children become more proficient and productive readers. When children first begin to read for meaning, their parents and teachers assist them in extracting information from the text and comprehending what it means. Kids replace such external monitors with self-monitoring as they improve as readers. They could ponder issues such as:

What will I learn from this, and why am I reading it?
Do I comprehend the information presented? (Examples include lists, alphabet books, and chapter books.)

What is the connection to what I already know?
Do the concepts and terms make sense to me, or do I need to pause and look them up or get clarification?

Reflection Time!

Self-Evalution			Daily Outcome
I Got It! ⬜	I Sort-of Got It! ⬜	I Didn't Got It YET! ⬜	

Demonstrate or Explain:

Name: _____   Date: _____

That is so motivating; now let me set my Ladder of Goals:

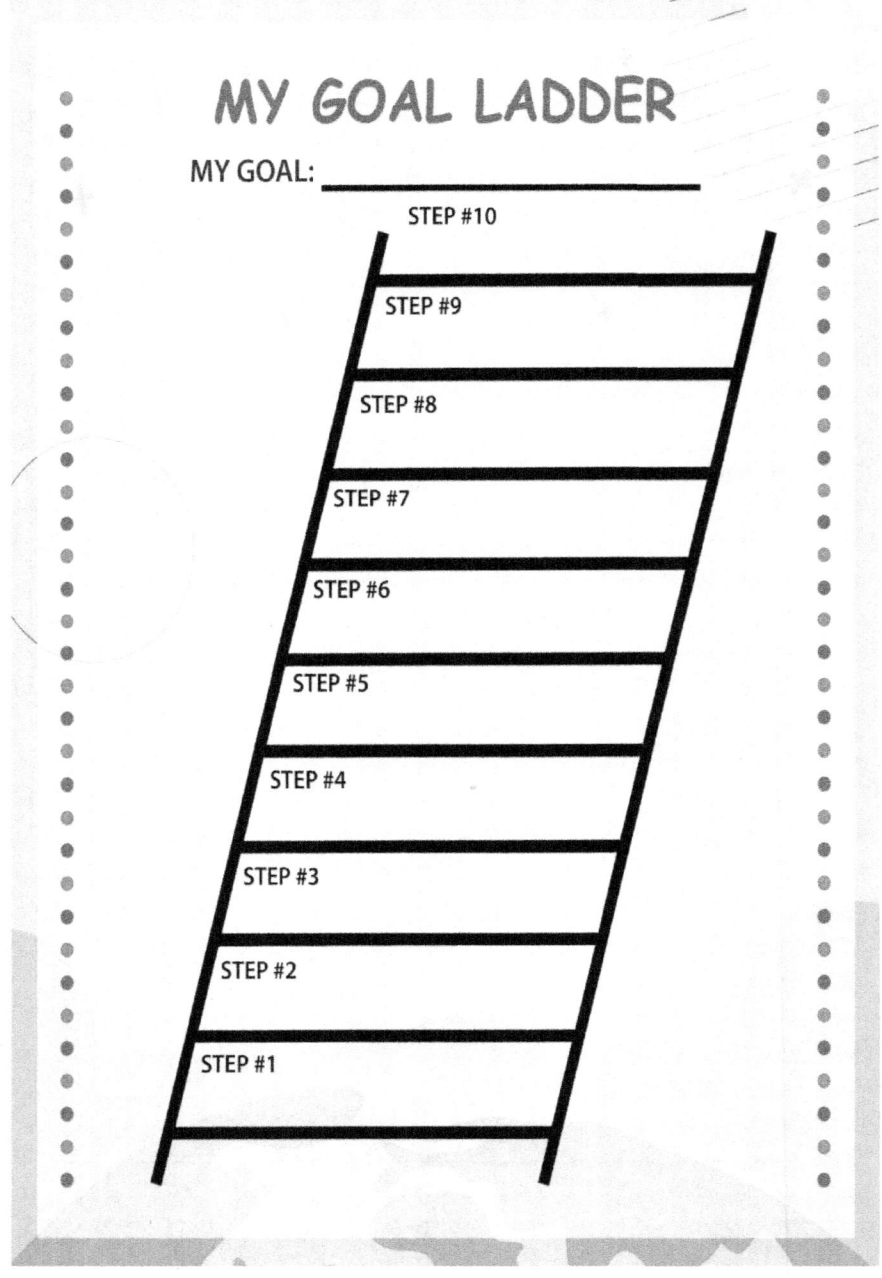

Chapter 5: Break the Negativity Loop

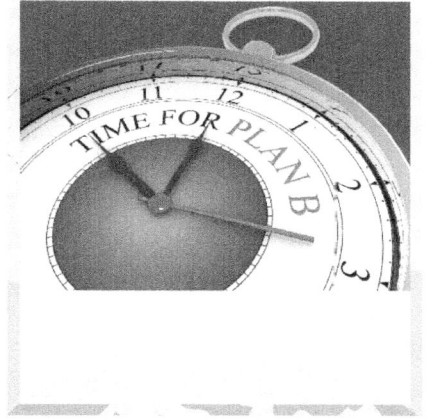

Children start to process negative thinking or negative thoughts when they hear "Don't do that," "You're breaking the rules," or "That's not right" from parents, caregivers, or teachers. We act as a kind of external regulator for them by offering advice.

In our lives, we've all come across "Negative Nancy" — those individuals who consistently anticipate the worst from every given circumstance.

Even though many of these individuals identify as "realists," there aren't many advantages to this pessimistic thinking style. This mentality is incredibly counterproductive during the relatively safe and shielded childhood period.

How, therefore, can we encourage a pessimistic child to have a more upbeat outlook on life?

It all comes down to comprehending where and how their negativity originates.

What Triggers your Anger ……

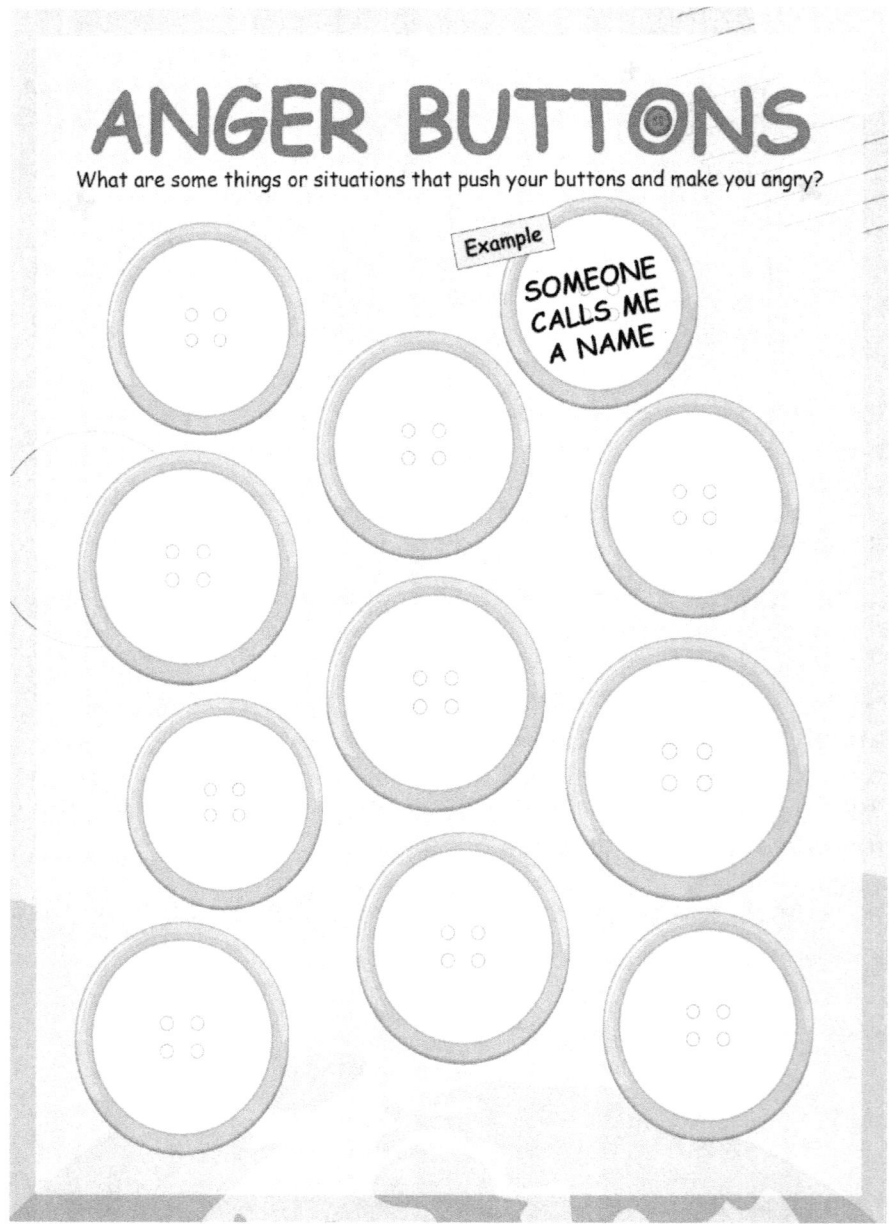

Why All the Discontent?

Numerous reasons can contribute to pessimism, which can also coincide with depressive or anxious symptoms. For the latter, criticizing a process or situation could be a defensive strategy or a way of "getting ready for the worst." While occasionally, this can be adaptable and successful. According to evolutionary psychology, our predecessors had a better chance of surviving if they constantly planned for the worst-case scenario. When a predator attacked in the past, there was a greater chance of suffering a severe injury or death. However, this tactic is useless for today's kids because the risks are much lower.

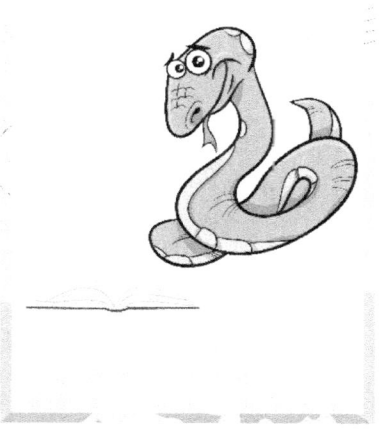

To figure out why your kids are acting so negatively and where it comes from, start by talking to them.

Ask inquiries like:

What could go wrong?

Why are you so confident in how events will pan out?

Why would hoping for the best rather than the worst be bad?

- **Observe and Hear**

To help their kids overcome negative thinking, parents must first listen to them, see how they handle their anxieties, and discuss their strengths. Watch them while they think. Ruminating was not the same as reflecting. A frightened hamster wheel is in motion while you ruminate. The same notion repeatedly surfaces, but it is never rephrased or viewed from a different perspective.

Negatively inclined children will occasionally say that they are sure they won't perform well on a school assignment or in a sporting event. Other times, people may avoid a situation or attempt a task even if they know they will fail.

- **Recognize and Rephrase**

Parents must take action if their children verbally or physically demonstrate those feelings. Recognize that they are concerned about performing well on a test or activity. Simply expressing one's emotions can increase a child's sense of self-awareness. They suddenly say, "I think I'm worried." Right from there, assist them in shifting their viewpoint.

Ask them a few questions to see if they can change their perspective or bring up history. "Say, 'I recall you were so nervous about taking that reading test last year, and you aced it. There was no issue. You can accomplish this.

Don't encourage your youngster to reject the views as you work to understand why they are harmful. Encourage them to see those negative thoughts as just one possibility among many.

> *"It's crucial to establish a family culture that accepts that failing is a necessary component of learning. In other words, both parents admit to making mistakes. We aren't ideal parents. We don't pretend to be ideal parents. We discuss our errors as they occur — for example when we blow a grant or make a mistake at work. We do not hide it. And when it does, we bring it out and say, "It happens to all of us; otherwise, we wouldn't be learning."* ***Johnson Miller***

- **Switch Your Attention**

A negative youngster could have a fixed mindset:

They hold the negative belief that their talent is fixed and unchangeable.

*However, this is not the case, which is why one of the oldest sayings in the book is **"practice makes you perfect"**!*

According to the growth mindset idea, we can "grow" in whatever way the process allows because we believe we can change and get better. In this sense, it favors highlighting the value of the process behind things rather than the final product.

Redirect your child's attention to things other than the outcome of a sporting event if they are feeling down about how they performed.

Other reasons why they engage in the sport?

They must be physically fit and healthy, develop their skills, and interact with their teammates. The advantages of the process much surpass the results of any given game. *'What you learn from each encounter, not whether you win or lose, get it right or wrong,'*

Here we go time to Change the Plan ……

My Change Plan

What behavior do I want to change?

☆ _____ ☆

What would happen if I no longer do this behavior?
_____

What can I do to start getting ready to change?

1. _____
2. _____
3. _____

What steps do I need to take to make these changes happen?

1. _____
2. _____
3. _____

What can others do to help me change my behavior?

1. _____
2. _____
3. _____

What will I know that I'm making progress?_____
_____

What can I do if I start going to my old behavior?
_____

What is something I can do today to start changing my behavior?_____
_____

5.1. Start with Validating Feelings

When you acknowledge your child's feelings of happiness, sadness, anger, or another strong emotion, you are validating those feelings for your child without passing judgment, placing expectations on them, or making remarks about what they "should" be experiencing instead. Validating is not repairing, correcting, imparting knowledge, or giving counsel.

Getting the "objective facts" regarding what made your child feel this way is less important for parents and other adults responsible for your children than making them feel seen, heard, and understood. Understanding the problem from your child's perspective and sharing an understanding of their experiences with them is necessary for validating your child's sentiments.

- **The significance of emotional validation**

Thanks to emotional validation, your children will learn it's okay to feel and express their feelings. Parents who show their children that it's normal to experience hurt, fear or, sadness occasionally serve as role models.

- **Dependable attachment and faith**

Additionally, it can increase trust between you and your child, fostering closer intimacy and a solid attachment. A youngster is reassured that they have a secure place to talk about and process their experience when they validate their experience. As children get older, this security can help them gain coping mechanisms and teach them to have confidence in themselves.

- **Emotional awareness**

Children's emotional intelligence can be developed through the advantages of emotional validation. Learning to pay attention to one's emotional moods helps a child's psychological development by promoting good emotional understanding.

- **Emotional control**

Children can develop coping mechanisms for managing and expressing their emotions when emotional validation is combined with kind instruction and interactions with parents. Kids experience the same emotions as adults; however, many lack the linguistic ability to express what they need from their caregivers, which is why many kids act out in the form of outbursts, tantrums, and emotional deregulation. The more your child's feelings and emotions are acknowledged by parents and other caregivers when angry, the less likely they will misbehave.

I Love Me .... ♥ ♥ ♥

YOU-nique!

Being unique means that there are certain things about you that make you stand out! What are 10 positive things that make you unique and different from everyone else? This can include your special talents, traits, or experience that you've had!

1. _____
2. _____
3. _____
4. _____
5. _____
6. _____
7. _____
8. _____
9. _____
10. _____

5.2. The Three Varieties of Self-Control

Children must be able to control their thoughts, behaviors, and emotions. They need self-control, a trait that enables them to apply the brakes and deliberate before acting, to accomplish that.

Self-control is a characteristic of the executive function skill set. Kids gradually acquire these abilities. *Impulse control, emotional control, and movement control* are the three different types of self-control.

Every child experiences impulsive or overly emotional moments but it's a recurring issue for certain kids. Any one or many forms of self-control may be difficult for them. Find out more about the three different self-control types.

i. *Impulse Management*

It entails the capacity to pause and consider an action before taking it. Kids with better impulse control can consider the repercussions before cutting in front of others or darting into traffic without looking. A kid with self-control can think for a moment, "I could get in trouble, or I could get wounded," and then choose something else.

However, children who lack self-control frequently act without first thinking. They can have a lot of problems at school or home. They may find it challenging to establish friends because some young people may not appreciate their erratic behavior.

Children who lack impulse control could:

- *Say things quickly and without considering*
- *Act rashly and without hesitation*

- *Display aggression toward other children*
- *When upset, overreact*
- *Interrupt frequently, talk excessively, or use uninvited speech*
- *Not begin homework assignments until almost time for bed.*
- *Complete assignments quickly*
- *One day, abide by the rules; the next, don't*

ii. *Emotional Management*

The capacity to control emotions is known as emotional control. Most children can bounce back from minor disappointment or criticism as they age. They are not sidetracked or overtaken by their emotions.

However, children with trouble managing their emotions could find it difficult to move over a traumatic situation. Even a minor setback, such as dropping a game or performing poorly on an exam, qualifies. They overreact, and their negative moods could persist for a while. Some children find it challenging to moderate their positive feelings. They could become overexcited and struggle to decompress after becoming happy.

Children who lack emotional control could exhibit the following behaviors:

- ✓ *When things don't go their way, they quickly become frustrated and quit.*
- ✓ *Not able to take criticism well and can't control their emotions long enough to complete tasks (like homework)*
- ✓ *Struggle to maintain composure when someone bothers or upsets them,*
- ✓ *Overreact to little setbacks or difficulties*
- ✓ *When angry or delighted, react in a vast, loud way.*

iii.   Movement Management

The capacity to control when and how our body moves is known as movement control. Kids who possess this kind of self-control can stay still when necessary. They can respect other people's privacy because of it. Being able to control their mobility makes it much simpler for individuals to comply with requests, such as waiting in line or sitting through a meal. At some time, all children struggle to regulate their movements. You can't stay motionless when you're so excited and energized but most children eventually outgrow this restlessness. If a child's inability to regulate their movements persists, hyperactivity may be the cause.

Children who lack motor control could exhibit the following behaviors:

- ✓ *Excessive activity or restlessness*
- ✓ *Pace or engage in hand games*
- ✓ *Difficulty remaining motionless or inline*
- ✓ *They roam around to disrupt conversations and games. Even after being instructed to stop, run and shout*
- ✓ *While the instructor is speaking, get up and move around.*
- ✓ *Move so quickly that they collide with objects or persons*
- ✓ *Families and educators must communicate what they observe in the home and at school when children struggle with self-control.*

- *Resilience and Self-worth*

Children can develop self-esteem and a real emotional sense of reality through these coping mechanisms and the coping mechanisms required to deal with challenging situations. Children who receive emotional validation may feel more capable of navigating their emotions healthily and avoiding dangerous or unhealthy situations.

I have a Power Question.

Name: _____   Date: _____

Possible Quiz Question	Answer

5.3 Be Positive: Try Being Optimistic!

Positive self-talk has a variety of benefits, "*People appear to believe that having a negative outlook and being realistic go hand in hand.*" They believe the worst-case scenario is significantly more likely than the best-case scenario but in reality, this isn't the case at all!

While negativity can impair the performance, optimistic attitudes and affirmations can help it. Such as the mentalities of some most well-known and accomplished athletes.

Do you ever hear a basketball champion declare, "I'm going to play today"?

No!

In pre-game interviews, you hear them saying, "I'm going to win, I'm the champion, and I'm the best." And it's not just arrogance being expressed here (although there might be a little of that, too).

So because having self-assurance and using motivational language is essential, we have cheer squads for the same reason, too!

Additionally, "they have that mindset because the instant they experience any self-doubt, they might compromise their performance."

What if your child is attributing their negativity to an actual event (rather than one that they see or anticipate), such as persistently poor performance or team defeats in sports? Well, being down won't accomplish anything,

It's a defense mechanism, but it doesn't improve performance, and it's easy to get caught in a vicious loop where there's little room for improvement.

Therefore, if having a pessimistic attitude has been linked to poor performance, altering attitudes may also be the key to altering the results.

Ok so you are so Talkative, let's Talk Positive

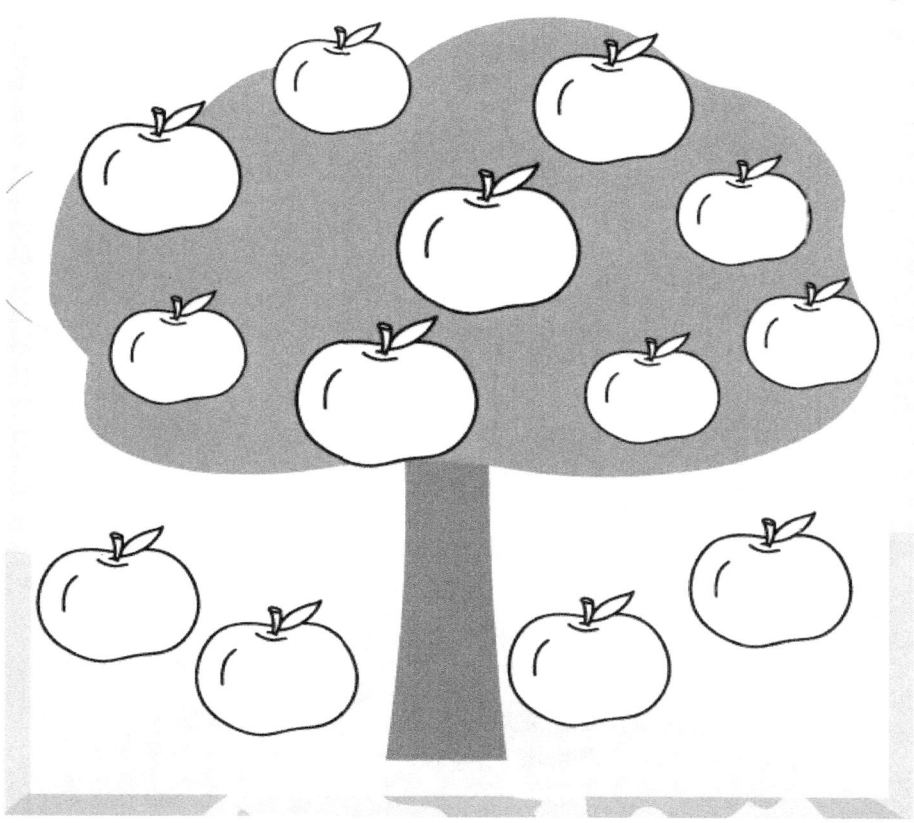

POSITIVE SELF TALK APPLE TREE

Write the positive things you say to yourself in the apples on the tree. In the apples that fell off the tree (the rotten apples) write the negative things you say to yourself.

POSITIVE SELF-TALK WHEEL

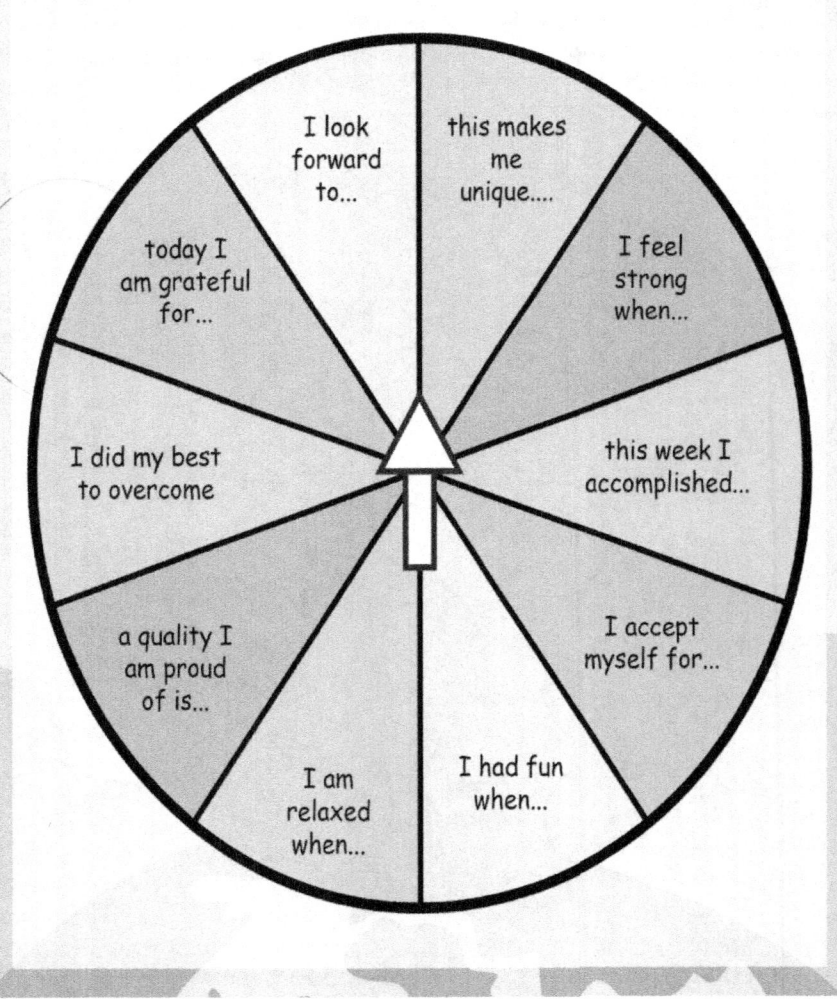

Discuss with your Parent or Friend and fill out your Positive Talk Chart

Name: _____ Date: _____ Class: _____

Blank Pie Chart with 24 Pieces

5.4. Develop

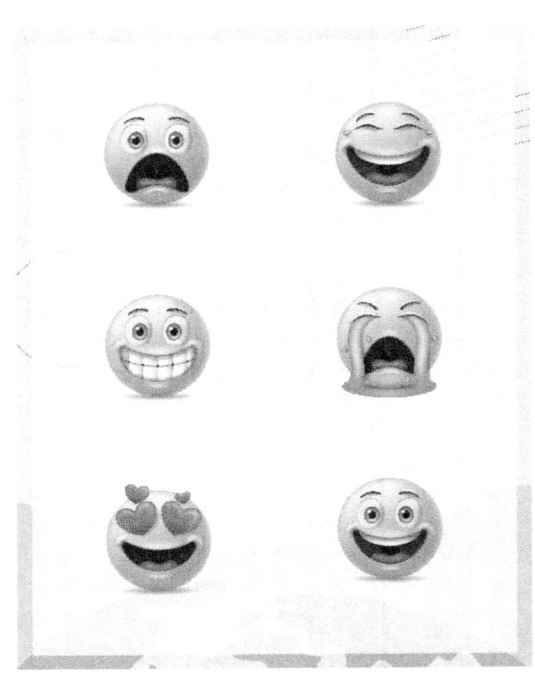

Thankfulness: *Practice Being Thankful*

It has been demonstrated that feeling grateful significantly affects our level of happiness.

That makes sense - the more appreciative we are of what we have, the less we think about what we lack. Higher levels of happiness and life satisfaction follow from this!

Talking with your negative child every day about the wonderful things that occurred, no matter how minor or insignificant they may appear, will help them learn to be thankful.

It might have been a simple, tasty treat they enjoyed at lunch, a fun play session they had with friends, or a fascinating new concept they studied in class. A specific approach to stop persistent negativity in its tracks is to put your attention on the positive aspects of life. So, in conclusion, while working with a pessimistic child:

- *Practice using constructive self-talk.*
- *Instead of focusing on results, consider processes.*
- *Promote an attitude of thankfulness.*

It's also critical to recognize that negativity is merely an adaptive or protective personality feature rather than a harmful one. It only takes addressing the cause of negativity and developing strategies to counter it to realize that many negative kids are pretty intelligent and conscientious.

If you discover that putting these ideas into practice has no discernible impact on your child's attitude, think about other potential causes, such as anxiety or depression, and think about seeking more assistance from a licensed psychologist.

The foundational elements of executive functioning: No other building blocks are pertinent because executive functioning is the foundational ability for many other developmental domains. However, there are several significant essential ideas that all parents and caregivers need to be aware of to build executive functioning skills.

5.5 Practical Approach and Frequently Asked Questions

Let's dig deeper...How can I know if my child has executive functioning issues?

Symptoms of executive functioning issues in children include:

- *Having trouble making goals.*

- *Show little understanding of the steps taken to make things happen.*
- *Have trouble getting a task going.*
- *Live in the now and don't consider the future or the implications.*
- *Unable to use past experiences to make plans renders disciplining methods ineffective.*
- *Even when it is useless, stick with the same approach when solving a recurring issue.*
- *Change abruptly from impulsive to rigid, frequently when anxiety levels rise.*
- *Possess trouble adjusting to change.*
- *Rarely adopt a strategy for a given situation.*
- *Have unreasonable expectations of their talents and low self-esteem.*
- *Having trouble suppressing their emotions long enough to act responsibly.*
- *Find the cause of their problems that are not under your control.*
- *Possess a low threshold for failure.*
- *Skip steps in a process become perplexing when the intended result is not achieved.*
- *Have trouble understanding that a task has sub-goals or ordering a series of stages.*
- *Have trouble changing viewpoints.*
- *Need to be reminded to keep others' sentiments in mind.*
- *Miss the "full picture" of a work or circumstance.*

What other issues can arise when a youngster struggles with executive functioning?

Children who struggle with executive functioning issues may also struggle with the following:

- **Behavior:** The child's actions, typically in response to their surroundings or the demands of their tasks.
- **Self-regulation:** is the capacity to achieve, maintain, and modify one's emotions, behavior, attention, and activity level in a socially acceptable way for a task or setting.
- **Social skills:** The ability to negotiate with others, understand and adhere to social standards, and participate in reciprocal engagement (verbally or nonverbally) are all examples of social skills.
- **Academic performance:** is how easily a student can finish academic assignments.
- **Attention and concentration:** Consistent effort, performing tasks without interruption, and maintaining that effort long enough to complete the task.

How much can executive functioning be enhanced?

Provide the reasoning behind new abilities a youngster learns, or else they may feel like the preparation for a task was a waste of time.

- **List the steps:** Assist the youngster by outlining the steps needed for assignments in advance to make them less challenging and more doable.
- **Use aids:** Make use of instruments like alarm clocks in watches, computers, pads, and timers.

- **Visuals:** Create visual schedules and check them frequently throughout the day.
- **Give two different kinds of information:** As well as spoken directions, provide the youngster with written (or visual) instructions.
- **Make "to-do" lists and checklists:** While estimating the time needed for each task or to complete assignments, use checklists. For instance, a student's checklist might contain the following items:

> *Pull out a pencil and paper.*
> *Write your name.*
> *Write the due date.*
> *Read the instructions.*

- **Calendars:** can keep track of tasks, deadlines, and other activities.
- **Improve the child's working environment:** by helping them organize their workspace and reduce clutter.
- **Teacher meetings:** Schedule regular meetings with a teacher or supervisor to discuss work and address issues.

Create routines: to help you reinforce your skills and recall the tasks at hand.

Here are some games to make you more Executive....

10 GAMES
TO IMPROVE
Executive Functioning Skills

1 — **BLURT** (self-control, metacognize)

2 — **SCRABBLE** (planning, organization)

3 — **PICTIONARY** (flexibility, time management)

4 — **DISTRACTION** (working memory, attention)

5 — **5 SECOND RULE** (time management, task initiation)

6 — **FREEZE** (self-control, attention)

7 — **JENGA** (self-control, flexibility, planning)

8 — **BRAINTEASERS** (perseverance, flexibility)

9 — **CHESS** (planning, flexibility, working memory)

10 — **SODUKU** (perseverance, working memory)

Which exercises can enhance *Executive Function*?

Multiple-step cut-and-paste projects that call for sequential completion of tasks are required and to help the youngster write down ideas strategically, use mind mapping.

- *Games:* Puzzles and games that require planning and problem-solving, such as "Go Getter" (River & Road game).
- ***Use lotus diagrams:*** *to help the youngster organize their thoughts on paper while setting clear guidelines for how much to write.*
- *When creating blocks, have the kid reproduce the designs from a 2D or 3D model.*
- *Drawing:* Use a model to draw an image. Next, create a partially completed replica of the same image and ask the youngster to complete it so that it resembles the model.
- ***Set goals with the youngster:*** *(e.g., help the child set attainable goals that are well-defined). Dissect objectives into manageable steps and discuss potential solutions with the youngster.*
- *Play games like 'Memory':* "I went to the shops and got a..." demanding the youngster recollect information.
- *Multitasking:* To help the youngster learn to switch from one activity to another, practice performing several tasks simultaneously. It may be beneficial to number the tasks.

Why should I go for therapy if I have executive functioning issues?

Therapeutic assistance for a child's executive functioning is crucial to:

- *Reduce the adverse behavioral effects of stress and anxiety.*

- *Give them the chance to acquire the fundamental abilities to make academic success easier.*
- *Make life easy for everyone in the family because when a youngster cannot deal with change, it can negatively impact everyone in the family and make daily tasks challenging, if not impossible.*
- *The earlier executive functioning issues are addressed, the simpler it is to implement change.*
- *Executive function is a scholarly ability, and different people require different amounts of modeling and support. They won't be able to acquire these skills without the proper direction.*

What are the consequences of untreated executive functioning issues?

Children who struggle with executive functioning may also struggle with the following:

- *Making friends and low sense of self.*
- *Unable to handle the responsibilities of life or school.*
- *Poor organizational and work habits.*
- *Losing track of personal items quite frequently.*
- *Poor academic performance.*
- *Not finishing everyday tasks, such as chores or schoolwork, promptly.*
- *Grandiose goals that they aspire to achieve but are unable to accomplish realistically.*

Let's Brainstorm

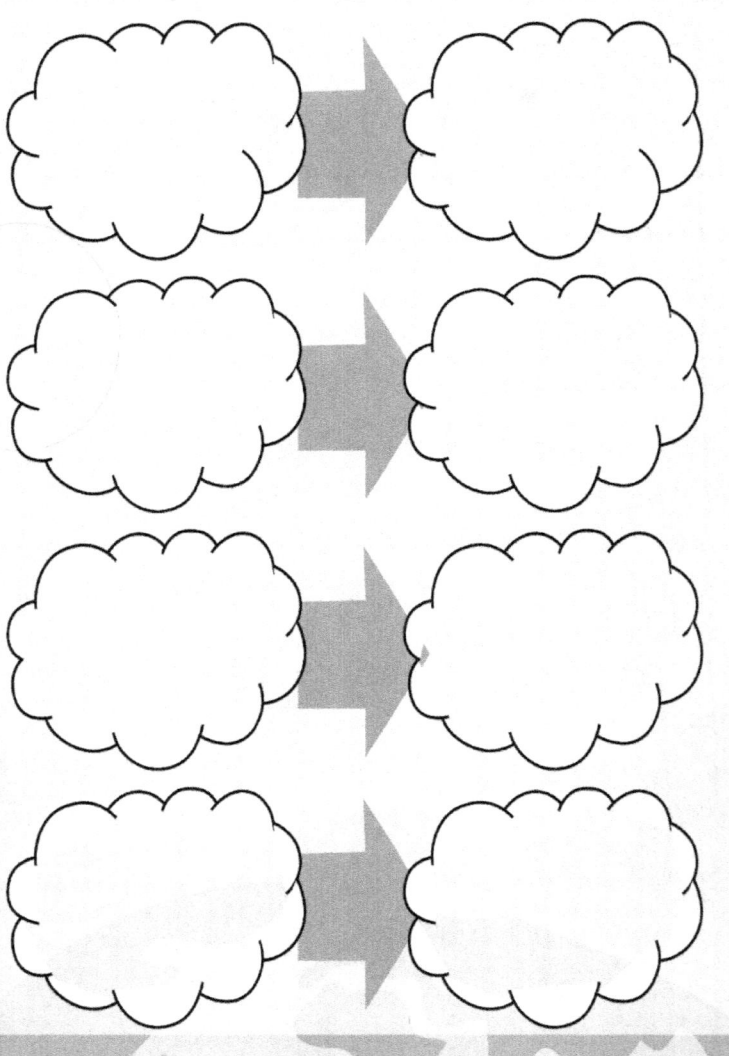

Outcomes

Success requires imagination, flexibility, self-control, and discipline. Fundamental executive functions include focusing, responding deliberately instead of impulsively, and mentally experimenting with ideas. Numerous activities, including computerized training, non-computerized games, and mindfulness activities improve children's executive functions. All successful programs necessitate regular practice and gradually increase the demands for executive function. Early executive-function training may help to prevent future achievement gaps from becoming more prominent since these activities are particularly advantageous to children with worse executive functions.

Like other developmental milestones, there is some normal variance in how quickly children reach executive function milestones. However, some children experience more significant challenges or delays in developing their executive function skills as compared to their peers or siblings.

Some kids' executive function issues include impulse control, outbursts, and emotional self-regulation. Some people might struggle more than others with organization, recalling directions, and understanding the classroom rules. It might be challenging for teenagers with executive function difficulties to develop independence and make long-term plans.

Contrary to popular assumption, executive functioning refers to various skills and does not develop linearly. The primary components of executive functions include inhibition control, or the ability to control impulses; working memory, a type of short-term memory that entails temporarily storing and manipulating information; and cognitive flexibility, or shifting attention (the ability to switch between thinking about different topics). With development spurts and opportunities for intervention, each of these skills develops at a distinct rate.

Environmental factors like childhood development trauma, family dynamics, and educational opportunity can considerably enhance or impede executive function skills. Fortunately, this implies how they can be significantly improved and adjusted. According to extensively researched evidence-based interventions, structured educational, neuropsychological, and socio-emotional programs can help children's executive functions.

Let's Conclude

Name: _____ Date: _____

Learning Frame

Today I learned about _____ with my freinds.

The tricky part is _____,

But it helps when I _____.

It's important that i know this because _____
_____
_____

Printed in Great Britain
by Amazon